I0412821

# IBS Diet Guide for the Novice

## Reduce Pain and Control IBS Symptoms with Diet

By: David P Fry

# PUBLISHERS NOTES

**Disclaimer**

This publication is intended to provide helpful and informative material. It is not intended to diagnose, treat, cure, or prevent any health problem or condition, nor is intended to replace the advice of a physician. No action should be taken solely on the contents of this book. Always consult your physician or qualified health-care professional on any matters regarding your health and before adopting any suggestions in this book or drawing inferences from it.

The author and publisher specifically disclaim all responsibility for any liability, loss or risk, personal or otherwise, which is incurred as a consequence, directly or indirectly, from the use or application of any contents of this book.

Any and all product names referenced within this book are the trademarks of their respective owners. None of these owners have sponsored, authorized, endorsed, or approved this book.

Always read all information provided by the manufacturers' product labels before using their products. The author and publisher are not responsible for claims made by manufacturers.

**Digital Edition**

# WHAT YOU WILL LEARN IN THIS BOOK

## How This Book Will Help You and Why

Are you or someone you know affected by Irritable Bowel Syndrome (IBS)? If that is the case and you want to learn more information about the condition then this book is perfect. Apart from providing a definition of what IBS is it also explains what the signs and symptoms are and then goes into the main focus of the book which is the diet that can help to alleviate the symptoms of the condition.

The book also outlines the foods that should not be included in the diet. It can be an extremely uncomfortable condition to deal with and persons that are afflicted will find the book extremely helpful.

Dive Right into the Book! Or Learn a Bit More About the Author

# TABLE OF CONTENTS

# DEDICATION

The book is dedicated to my Aunt Fiona. She has been fighting the negative effects of IBS for years and through her strength and her will to find a viable solution for herself I got the drive to do my own research. Without her this book would not have been created.

# CHAPTER 1- WHAT IS IBS AND HOW DOES IT AFFECT AN INDIVIDUAL?

If you, or someone you love, has been diagnosed with irritable bowel syndrome, you may be wondering exactly what is irritable bowel syndrome, and what you can do about it. In this chapter, we offer a short explanation about what irritable bowel syndrome is, how it is diagnosed, and how you can manage it if you have it.

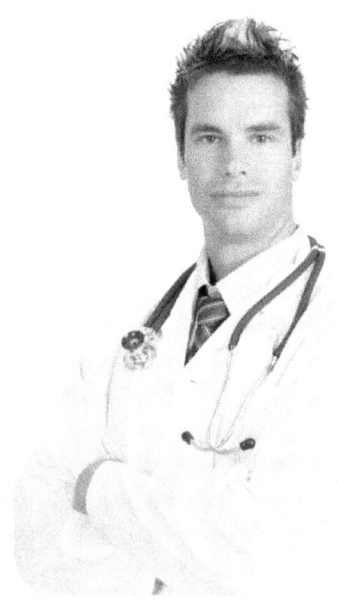

**So What Is Irritable Bowel Syndrome?**

IBS, or irritable bowel syndrome, is actually a fairly common digestive tract disorder, that does not cause permanent damage, but that can be painful and uncomfortable.

There are actually three distinct types of IBS – some sufferers have constipation mainly, some have diarrhea mainly, and others have a combination of the two. All types are usually accompanied by abdominal pain, bloating and sometimes excess gas.

Irritable Bowel Syndrome, or IBS as it is often referred too, has seen a dramatic increase over the last 10 years. IBS has become increasingly widespread in the developed countries of the world and is now considered the most common digestive disorder, accounting for over 50% of visits to gastro-enterologists.

**What Are Irritable Bowel Syndrome Triggers?**

Some people find that stress can trigger a bout of IBS, or start it off entirely. Others find that specific foods cause them to suffer symptoms, while hormones can trigger IBS in women, usually in sync with their menstrual cycle. Some people may have a combination of these symptoms, or some may find that their symptoms appear after a bout of illness.

**How Is IBS Diagnosed?**

IBS is usually only diagnosed if you have suffered the 'classic' symptoms mentioned above for some time. It is typically a chronic disease, and if your symptoms have just started, without a specific cause or reason, then your doctor might suspect something else is the cause. In that case, he or she will probably test for those other diseases or disorders; as thus far, there is no concrete test for IBS.

**How Is IBS Treated?**

The best method of treat IBS is to take a holistic approach. Diet should be addressed, as should lifestyle. Persons with IBS should avoid stress as much as possible, and they should try to figure out what their triggers are, in terms of both food, and lifestyle factors.

Thankfully, IBS is not something that gets worse throughout your life. The symptoms are usually the same per individual. In fact, some people's irritable bowel syndromes calms down on its own, though that Is not something you should count on for yourself. You might be one that will need to actively seek treatment all your life.

One reason that many people seem to get IBS is for stress related reasons. Simply de-stressing your life can take away all of the symptoms you are experiencing. Try going out for a relaxing massage or take a long weekend as a vacation.

Beyond that, there are some foods that are known to make IBS symptoms worse for some people. These foods might make you gassy or are just not easily digestible. Try to keep a record of the things you eat so you can chart which foods seem to peak your symptoms.

If those things are not your cure for IBS it might be necessary to take some medication to make your symptoms better. Your doctor can advise you whether or not you need a specific prescription or if over the counter medications instead. Also, remember that the first thing you try might not be what ultimately works for you.

Trying to cure IBS might take years to figure out. The good news is that you have already decided to take active steps to make your life better. That means that you will not have to suffer long because you will find what works best for you.

There are new developments being made in the medical community all the time. There may come a time when there is a cure available for irritable bowel syndrome sufferers. Until then, it's important to find one on your own.

**Irritable Bowel Syndrome Statistics**

The world has a growing problem when it comes to irritable bowel syndrome. If nothing else it is a warning to people that they need to pay attention to their bodies and treat them well because one day they could join the millions who suffer from it.

Worldwide, irritable bowel syndrome affects between 9-20% of the population, making it the most common gastrointestinal disorder. It is estimated that some 35 million Americans suffer from irritable bowel syndrome.

Although some people have such mild symptoms that they don't know they have IBS, physicians report it is still one of the most common disorders in patient visits. In the United States alone annually there are between 2.4-3.5 million physician visits for IBS.

Irritable bowel syndrome is the most common diagnosis to patients by gastroenterologists.

The total amount of money lost or spent because of IBS estimated around $21 billion annually. This is due to medical expenses, reduced productivity, and missed work.

Males account for 35-40% of people diagnosed with irritable bowel syndrome. While females account for 60-65%.

60% of IBS sufferers will develop Fibromyalgia. 70% of Fibromyalgia sufferers report having some symptoms of irritable bowel syndrome.

**IBS for Women Statistics**

Irritable Bowel syndrome is a more harmful disorder to women than it is to men.

Irritable bowel syndrome is most likely to occur during a woman's child bearing years with the most severe symptoms occurring during premenstrual and postovulatory phases.

IBS symptoms are more severe in women who suffer from it during menstruation while women IBS sufferers who become pregnant actually see improvements in symptoms.

Over 50% of patients complaining of lower abdominal pains when they go to the gynecologist actually suffer from irritable bowel syndrome.

Endometriosis is diagnosed much more often in women suffering from IBS than women who don't. Data also shows that women not suffering from IBS are three times less likely to get a hysterectomy than women who do.

Studies now show that IBS costs billions of dollars in visits to doctors, alternative practitioners, diagnostic testing and treatments.

IBS is the second most common cause of lost workdays after the common cold, not to mention lost social moments with friends and loved ones, spoilt nights out, a restrictive lifestyle and just feeling plain awful!

To put this major problem into perspective millions of people throughout the developed world including the USA, Britain, Australia and the European Union have their lives affected by IBS.

IBS affects children, teenagers, young adults, the middle-aged and the elderly.

Good Bowel health is increasingly seen as the cornerstone to general good health and the best immune system you can have against illness.

With statistics like these it's hard for anyone to try and ignore irritable bowel syndrome. Even if you don't currently have IBS there is always the chance that it will develop.

# Chapter 2- What are the Symptoms of IBS?

IBS symptoms can be extremely difficult to deal with. Many of them are so uncomfortable that you don't feel like you can live your life anymore. Do all you can to treat these symptoms and you'll be able to start feeling like yourself again.

The first thing to keep in mind is that just because you have some of the IBS symptoms does not mean that you have IBS. Your symptoms could signal a less severe problem or even a more severe problem.

That is why it's best to monitor the IBS symptoms. If something seems to be out of the ordinary for your body you should see your doctor. Your doctor will probably ask you many different questions and do different tests in order to make their diagnosis.

There are many different IBS symptoms to keep track of. This is because they show up differently in different people. Some of the more common ones are bloating, cramps, gas, diarrhea, and constipation. Another common one that many people don't consider is stress or anxiety.

Other symptoms related to IBS but are nongastrointestinal are:

Headache

Anxiety or depression

Fatigue

Backache

Unpleasant taste in the mouth

Heart palpitations (feeling like the heart skips a beat or is fluttering)

Sleeping problems (insomnia) not caused by symptoms of IBS

Sexual problems, such as pain during sex or reduced sexual desire

Urinary symptoms (urgent or frequent need to urinate, trouble emptying the bladder, trouble starting the urine stream)

All of these symptoms are most prominent in times of stress, after meals, and for women, during menstruation.

There are three classification types associated with irritable bowel syndrome symptoms:, or diarrhea-predominant symptoms

**IBS-D** which is associated with patients who suffer from primarily diarrhea related symptoms

**IBS-C** which is associated with patients who suffer from primarily constipation related symptoms

**IBS-A** which is associated with patients who suffer from alternating symptoms between diarrhea constipation

Curing symptoms of each classification may be different patient to patient and it is good to find a program that works for an individual's needs. Try to keep a record of the IBS symptoms that you experience. Mark down when they occur and how long they last. When you do this, it becomes a lot easier to discuss the condition and any possible treatments with your doctor. Make sure that you're making every effort to get to know your symptoms.

The more you know about the way your body works, the better equipped you'll be to handle your symptoms as they come. You might have to try a variety of different treatment options in order to get rid of your IBS symptoms, but the results will be well worth it.

No one sets out with the hopes that they will get IBS. It happens to many people and can be confusing. It doesn't seem fair that others get to live an IBS free life and you're stuck with these symptoms for the rest of yours.

Even so, be thankful that there are treatment options for your IBS symptoms. Do everything you can do in your power to make sure that you don't become a slave to this condition. Your symptoms don't have to ruin your life.

# CHAPTER 3- IBS TREATMENT OPTIONS

Irritable bowel syndrome (IBS) can put a damper on many activities in your life. Having uncomfortable symptoms is a problem that you'll definitely want to eliminate as much as possible. The best thing for you to do is to find an IBS treatment that will work for you.

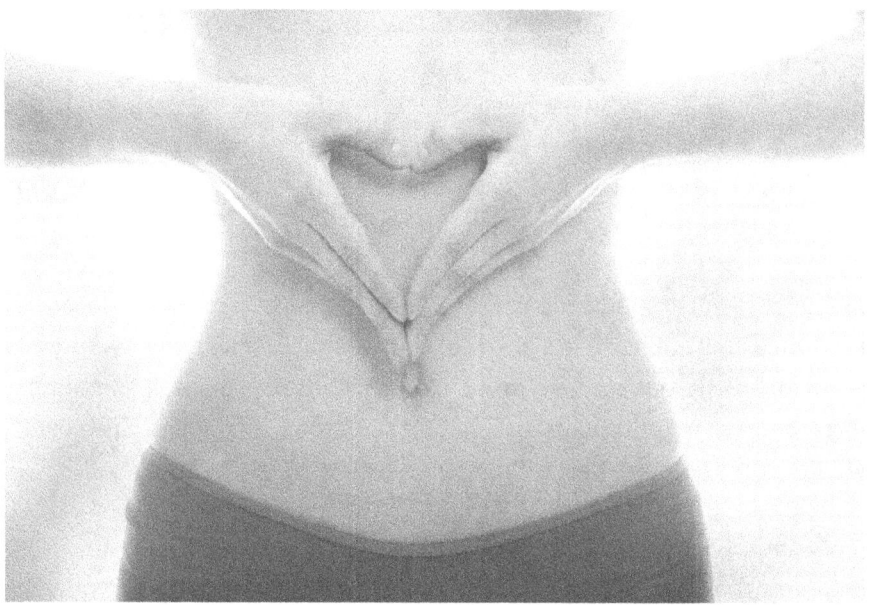

The first thing to note is that IBS is a chronic condition. That means that you will likely be dealing with it for the rest of your life. Some people experience much more severe symptoms than others, and the severity will often determine the treatment that you need.

Also, make sure that any treatment plan you start is given the thumbs up by your doctor. They are the best ones to make sure that your IBS treatment is the best option for you.

There are certain steps and guidelines that are usually followed for an irritable bowel syndrome treatment.

1. You will need to figure out what triggers your IBS. This can be anything from different foods to stressors in your life. Once you know what triggers your IBS, you can take steps to avoid these activities or actions.

2. There are several things that IBS sufferers have in common. Some triggers seem to be fairly universal. Try to avoid fatty foods, caffeine, alcohol, and gassy foods.

3. Make sure that you get plenty of exercise; try jogging or walking around your neighborhood. Getting this movement can help to stimulate your bowels so that they are not as uncomfortable.

4. There are also medications that you might take as an irritable bowel syndrome treatment. These medications tend to reduce your symptoms. Remember, there is no cure for IBS. You might take things like Imodium, Paxil, or Elavil in order to reduce certain symptoms or triggers. Speak with your doctor about the best option for you.

5. Reduce your stress. Try finding things that you like to do and feel comfortable doing. If you know that something is going to cause you a lot of anxiety, try your best to get through it or avoid it altogether.

Finding an irritable bowel syndrome treatment can take some trial and error. There are many people who have this condition and do find relief for their symptoms. Do everything you can to find the right treatment for you so that you can start to live your life again.

It is also important to note that many people who develop IBS start to feel a bit of depression and/or anxiety. This is one of the worst symptoms and can have a large impact on your daily life and interactions. Finding and irritable bowel syndrome cure becomes absolutely essential for these people. In this case, your doctor might prescribe an anti-depression or anti-anxiety medication.

If your IBS is ruining your life or stopping your enjoyment of certain activities you need to take action. Even if you can't ultimately cure IBS there are many things you can do to lead as normal a life as possible; do everything you can to monitor your disease and figure out what makes you feel worse and what will make you feel better.

There is no irritable bowel syndrome cure, but there are many things you can do to decrease the toll it takes on your life. Start finding your regimen today.

Your doctor may recommend specific medications to treat your IBS. He or she may recommend an antidepressant to help alleviate the symptoms of IBS because there is a link between depression and abdominal pain. If you are not clinically depressed the anti depressant medication in low doses may still help because it will inhibit the neurons that control the intestines.

More IBS treatments that can be helpful are antibiotics and counseling. If your doctor suspects your abdominal symptoms are caused by bacteria in the bowel, he may prescribe antibiotics. However, you should never insist that your doctor prescribe an antibiotic just because you think it will help. Taking too many antibiotics will do more harm than good. If you have a lot of stress in your life then you may benefit from professional counseling to help you deal with your stress. IBS symptoms will become worse with stress.

There are things you can do at home to reduce your symptoms of IBS. First of all, eat a healthy diet that contains plenty of fruits and vegetables. This will increase the fiber in your diet. Make sure you are drinking enough water. A good colon cleansing can help also. When you cleanse the colon of old fecal matter and toxins, you will restore the normal function of your colon.

As you can see you have a few options when it comes to IBS treatments. When you get your irritable bowel symptoms under control, you will be able to enjoy life again.

# CHAPTER 4- REVIEW OF MEDICATIONS RECOMMENDED FOR IBS

If you suffer from IBS this can help; independent research has been conducted looking for natural treatments that can help you control your irritable bowel syndrome. Customer testimonials have been researched in addition to keeping abreast of industry news.

The medications below are typically recommended as courses of treatment for IBS:

**Serovera**

Serovera Amp 500 is a natural supplement that is formulated specifically for those who suffer from gastrointestinal inflammation and irritable bowel syndrome.

Serovera claims to take a fresh approach to combating intestinal disorders and autoimmune diseases. It does this by providing a supplement that is natural and non-toxic. This supplement is safe enough to take every day for a long period of time. Serovera claims that 98% of the people that take their supplement have a significant improvement in their health.

**Usability of Serovera**

The number of capsules you take are dependent upon the severity of your symptoms. For those with severe gastrointestinal symptoms such as IBS it is recommended that you start with three capsules first thing in the morning on an empty stomach. On day two, you will increase to five capsules in the morning. On day three, you will take five capsules in the morning and four capsules in the evening before going to bed. You will remain at nine capsules a day until all of your symptoms subside. Then continue with nine capsules a day for thirty more days. After the thirty days, the maintenance dose of Serovera is three capsules daily.

## Serovera Customer Feedback

During our research, we asked the question, "Does Serovera work or is it a scam?" Our research found that customers who used Serovera noticed an improvement in their symptoms after about a month. Once the symptoms improve, the maintenance dose of three capsules per day kept the pain and diarrhea under control. Most customers continue to use Serovera for a lifetime.

## Serovera Guarantee

Serovera will give a full refund on any unopened bottle of the produce within 90 days. You must send the receipt of purchase along with unopened products. Serovera will refund your money with no questions asked.

## Overall Opinion of Serovera AMP 500 For IBS Relief

This product is extracted and freeze dried from the aloe vera plant. The great thing about this product is it is 100% certified organic. It does not contain toxins, and it will not conflict with other medications. It produces no side effects, and it is safe for long term use. The website is easy to navigate and this company offers a strong money back guarantee. The products have been lab certified to guarantee the authenticity of the product's ingredients.

## Digestrol

Digestrol is a dietary supplement that contains a combination of natural herbs and other ingredients that you can't get in your diet. These ingredients have been proven to provide digestive support and alleviate the symptoms of irritable bowel syndrome.

**Digestrol Claims and Benefits**

Digestrol claims it can alleviate the symptoms of gastrointestinal distress caused by the typical western diet. The natural dietary supplement not only alleviates symptoms of the lower bowel such as diarrhea, gas and bloating it will also relieve upper gastrointestinal symptoms such as heartburn and upset stomach.

Because this supplement is formulated from natural ingredients, you can use it for the rest of your life without worrying about negative side effects.

**Usability of Digestrol**

This product comes in easy to swallow tablets. You can follow the instructions on the bottle for the recommended dosage. Some people have been able to adjust the amount of pills they take each day according to their symptoms.

**Digestrol Customer Feedback**

During our research, we asked the question, "Does Digestrol work or is it a scam?" Our research found that those who have used Digestrol as directed have found relief from many various gastrointestinal symptoms. Some people claim to have relief after the first dose. Those who use Digestrol long term report normal digestive function.

## Digestrol Guarantee

Digestrol offers a complete satisfaction 90 day money back guarantee. They want you to give the product some time to work so they do not accept returns less than 30 days from the purchase date. But after 30 days, if you are not happy with the product you can return the product for a refund.

## Overall Opinion of Digestrol For IBS Relief

The active ingredients in Digestrol have been supported by substantiated research found in major publications such as the National Institute of Health and the National Library of Medicine. Since this product is made from natural supplements, it is gentle to your system while being extremely effective for IBS sufferers.

## Bowtrol

Bowtrol colon control is an all natural product that has been developed for people with a sensitive colon. The ingredients found in this product will calm the digestive tract and help to alleviate the annoying symptoms of irritable bowel syndrome.

## Bowtrol Claims and Benefits

Bowtrol claims that it does more than just eliminate the occasional bouts of diarrhea that accompany IBS. It claims that it supports the nutritional balance in your body by protecting and strengthening the lining of the intestinal tract.

The benefit of a healthy intestinal tract is the proper absorption of nutrients from the foods you eat. When your body is able to absorb the proper nutrients you will have more energy and look and feel healthier.

## Usability of Bowtrol Colon Control

This product comes in easy to swallow capsules. You should take two to four capsules in the morning and two to four capsules at night. If your diarrhea continues you can increase this dosage by one capsule at a time until your symptoms subside.

## Bowtrol Colon Control Customer Feedback

During our research, we asked the question, "Does Bowtrol Colon Control work or is it a scam?" Our research found that people who used Bowtrol colon control for their IBS symptoms found some relief within twenty four hours and significant relief from their symptoms with continued long term use.

## Bowtrol Colon Control Guarantee

Bowtrol takes great pride in the superior quality of their products, and they strive to make the customer happy. You may return any unused and unopened product within 90 days for a money back refund.

## Overall Opinion of Bowtrol Colon Control

Bowtrol is a company that has been around since 2002. They are a member of the Natural Products Association, and they strive to provide premium quality health and beauty products made from only the finest all natural ingredients. Bowtrol claim the ingredients found in Bowtrol Colon Control have been proven to work for IBS, and they are safe. This product is competitively priced, however we did find some negative reviews as well as testimonials from satisfied customers.

# CHAPTER 5- WHAT IS THE IBS DIET AND WHO IS IT SUITED FOR?

Pain, bloating, diarrhea and constipation...If you are an IBS sufferer, these symptoms are probably an everyday thing for you. Often getting rid of IBS seems to be almost as difficult and tiresome as the suffering and pain we have to go through. The good news is that IBS doesn't have to be with us for the rest of our lives. If I was able to get rid of it by following a properly constructed irritable bowel diet plan, so will you.

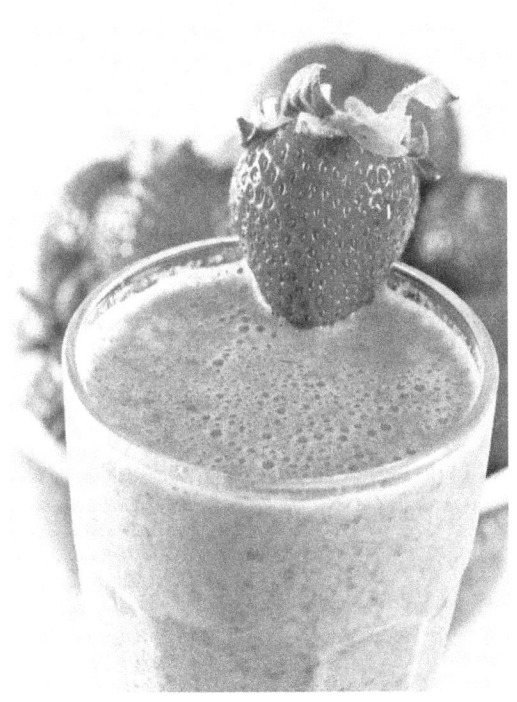

Before I tried it, I visited quite a few doctors and spent money on expensive treatments that worked only partially. Being fed up with it, I decided to dig deeper and find out as much as I could about my condition. I read a lot about nutrition for IBS and found out that a good diet for irritable bowel syndrome was really a necessity in order to get rid of IBS once and for all. I even started putting together a diet plan of my own but I gave up halfway – there were just too many things I still didn't know about to make it work. And then, pretty much incidentally, I stumbled across a great program.

What made me feel skeptical about it was the fact that the program's creator claims that you can actually eat most of your favorite foods. When I read the whole book and learned about the few simple principles I was supposed to follow, however, it all started to look quite convincing. The thing that I really liked about the program was the great selection of recipes that looked surprisingly yummy. All of this convinced me to give this IBS diet plan a try.

After just a few of days I noticed a decrease in the usual intensity of my IBS symptoms and after a month I was shocked to see an improvement that was way beyond what I had expected...After over a year of following the program's principles I can honestly say that my IBS is gone for good.

As much as I believe in the principles of the IBS diet, however, I have to warn you that this is not some sort of a magic cure. It is a well researched nutrition plan that can really improve your health but only as long as you stick to it. Think about a person that lost a significant amount of weight because he or she was following a proper diet. Would that person maintain the lower weight if he or she decided to go back to the old eating habits? The same applies to any irritable bowel diet plan.

I hope that my story will encourage you to make the necessary changes in your diet. If you do, it will have a dramatic effect on not only your IBS symptoms, but your entire health.

**Irritable Bowel Syndrome Diet Tips**

If you suffer from IBS you may want to learn how you can control the problem through alterations in the type of food that you consume. There are a number of irritable bowel syndrome diet tips that have been shown to produce positive results.

The actual cause of IBS is still not fully known. The reason why the intestines become so badly affected can be due to various reasons; each of us has a different metabolism. There are people who can eat any type of food with no negative effect and others that have problems with a wide variety of foods. If your colon is sensitive then you will need to make changes in your diet to stop flare ups.

Even though most of us lead very busy lives it is still essential to devote an adequate amount of time to eating correctly and more so if you have been diagnosed with IBS.

A healthy diet for irritable bowel sufferers does not have to be flavorless. There are a range of tasty and delicious foods that can be taken without causing a problem for your intestines. For example a typical balanced diet should include natural juices such as grape or cranberry, snacks such as bananas and crackers, lots of salad, and an evening meal that contains a small portion of meat alongside pasta or rice.

The main principle in an IBS diet is to remove the substances that can cause irritation; this includes all junk food and processed foods. Even alcohol, sodas, dairy, and chocolate should not be consumed at all.

To find out the exact irritable bowel diet that you should consume along with actual menus for different days it can be useful to find a solid resource on IBS diet. There you will be given you a shopping list of all the foods that are right for your condition.

**Irritable Bowel Diet – It's all About Finding the Right Balance**

If you have recently been diagnosed with irritable bowel syndrome then you may feel rather concerned. It is an illness that affects the digestion system, specifically the intestines and colon. If you have IBS then you will frequently have episodes of diarrhea, stomach cramps, bloating and gas. There is medication available that can control the symptoms to a small degree, but health experts suggest that an individual with IBS should consume a special irritable bowel diet that contains foods which are known to not cause an irritation in the gut.

To begin with you will need to increase the amount of fiber that you consume on a daily basis. By eating a lot of fiber your bowel movements will be more regularized and this will result in less stomach pain. Fiber is present in brown bread and brown rice, fruits, vegetables, and cereal. Of course it takes time for a high fiber diet to work its magic, don't expect to see results in one or two days.

A health specialist will also recommend that an IBS sufferer also cuts out certain foods from their lives. This should definitely include any junk food or other items that contain a lot of saturated fats. Spicy food should also be removed as this can cause an irritation in the lining of the intestine. Dairy and red meats should also be drastically cut back as should all types of sodas.

The best irritable bowel syndrome diet is always going to be a balanced one. Make sure you eat enough fresh fruit and vegetables. If you feel you have to hectic a schedule to spend hours preparing healthy meals each day then try making juices or smoothies out of fruit and vegetables; this is often the best way to get our required intake of vitamins and minerals.

If you have tried making alterations to your diet and yet are still suffering from the symptoms of IBS then you should look for a professionally written irritable bowel diet plan containing a list of foods that will help you to regain a normal life.

# Chapter 6- What Foods Should NOT Be Included In the IBS Diet?

IBS affects many people, and we are often told that sticking to an IBS diet plan is one way to treat the debilitating symptoms that the disorder presents. However, there's no one size fits all diet plan that helps every sufferer of IBS, so in this chapter, we look at how to develop your own IBS diet plan, which should lessen the effect of symptoms of the disorder.

**Understanding Trigger Foods**

There are no hard and fast rules as to which foods will trigger your IBS symptoms, however, there are some foods and beverages that are known to trigger IBS in more people than not.

These foods include dairy products, chocolate, grains like wheat, cabbage, beans, caffeinated drinks, barley or rye, certain fruits and alcohol. Not everyone will react to all of them, and some people may only have one or two trigger foods. Some may have trigger foods that are not on the common list.

**Keep a Food Diary**

If you desire to find out if there are any foods on the list that constantly causes you to have an IBS flare up or if you have any other triggers which are not on this list, the best solution is to keep a food diary for two to three weeks. Record everything that you eat, as well as your reaction to it.

**Eliminate All the Triggers**

The most efficient method of determining if you are triggered by one of the common offenders in IBS is to remove all of them from your diet for a week and then reintroduce them one at a time, for a few days at a time. If you realize that you experience a negative reaction to that particular food during that period of time, and then you can identify it as a trigger, and if not, then it is probably safe. Continue doing this until you have worked through all the common triggers, as well as the ones you suspect from your food diary.

Once you have put together a list of foods that you always react to, it should be relatively easy to put together your own IBS diet plan. Simply leave out the foods that cause a reaction in you, and eat the foods that do not.

You may need to adjust your shopping list a little, and develop new recipes, or switch to a non-dairy or low gluten diet, but it should be well worth the effort.

Continue to monitor your progress on your IBS diet plan, and make a note when any new foods you try give you a bad reaction. By eliminating the foods that trigger constipation, diarrhea, gas or other symptoms, and only consuming the foods that you recognize are 'harmless' you should fundamentally eliminate your IBS symptoms over time.

IBS can be hard to manage, but if you stick to a diet that you know you can trust, that's half the battle won. Then just avoid stress, and remember to keep medication for bloating, diarrhea or cramping on hand, and you should find that IBS is a manageable condition.

According to doctors there really is no cure for IBS. It's like having a cold sore. The virus that cause the cold sore lives dormant in your system until something triggers the cold sore to appear. This trigger could be a certain food, hormones or stress. This same holds true for IBS. Once you discover you have irritable bowel syndrome you will always be susceptible to the symptoms. But luckily you can keep the symptoms under control when you learn what your triggers are.

# CHAPTER 7- IS COLON CLEANSING BENEFICIAL FOR IBS?

**Control IBS & Enjoy Your Food**

The next best thing to an IBS cure is to do a good colon cleansing. This will alleviate your irritable bowel symptoms because it cleanses your system of built up fecal matter and toxins. Once the lining of the colon is clean, it will be able to perform properly. When you search for a colon cleanser, look for one that has natural ingredients. This will be much easier on your system and not cause additional bloating or diarrhea.

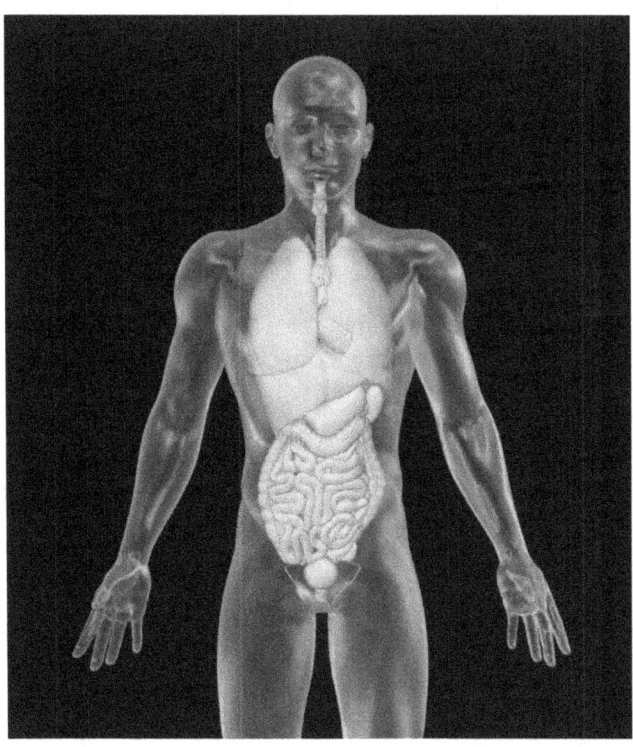

**The Benefits of Colon Cleansing**

**Improves the Way the Digestive System Works**

As the colon is cleansed, the waste that is undigested gets pushed through the system and it allows for the absorption of nutrients. If waste remains in the body for an extended period of time, it can lead to illness that occurs from the buildup of bacteria. When the colon is cleansed it gets rid of the unnecessary waste.

**Reduces the Instances of Constipation and Promotes Regularity**

Constipation is not something that persons enjoy especially when it occurs often. The digestive system is slow to respond and in the short term, the waste will stay in the body longer than it should. This will cause an increase in the possibility of harmful toxins getting into the blood. It can also trigger other illnesses and conditions like varicose veins and hemorrhoids.

**An Increase in Energy**

Getting rid of toxins from the body leaves the individual feeling refreshed ad it causes the energy that would be spent on trying to get the waste out to be used elsewhere. Persons that have gone through the process of colon cleansing have stated that they feel a boost in energy and that they sleep much more comfortably and have improved blood circulation.

**Increases the Absorption of Nutrients and Vitamins by the Body**

Only nutrients, vitamins and water are passed into the bloodstream from a clean colon. An unclean colon will push bacteria and toxins in to the bloodstream as well. As soon as the colon is clean there is no block to the passage of the essential nutrients and vitamins into the bloodstream.

**Enhances Concentration**

An inefficient diet coupled with the inadequate absorption of vitamins can cause an individual to have less focus and become easily distracted. The buildup of toxins and mucous in the colon can inhibit the body from functioning properly even if the diet is perfect. When the colon is cleansed it helps to improve focus and causes an improvement in overall health.

**Jumpstarts the Weight Loss Process**

Foods that do not contain a lot of fiber tend to go through the colon much more slowly than foods that are high in fiber. This causes an excess buildup of mucous which sticks to the walls of the intestines and triggers a buildup of fecal matter.

The process of colon cleansing can trigger the weight loss process. There are persons that state that they have lost up to a maximum of twenty pounds in just a month. Typically the colon weight approximately four pounds when it is empty and it can hold up to eight meals while the process of digestion occurs. The process of colon cleansing can help to speed up the metabolism.

**Lowers the Possibility of the Onset of Colon Cancer**

Everything that is consumed, inhaled and absorbed by the body will end up being processed by the liver and the gastrointestinal system. If these toxins remain in the system for an extended period of time, it can cause problems. When the waste is expelled from the body, it reduces the instances of cancerous growths, cysts and polyps growing in the gastrointestinal tract and colon.

There are a few other things you can do to relieve your IBS symptoms. Start eating several smaller meals throughout the day instead of larger meals. If you are convinced that stress is a trigger for your symptoms, try a few stress reduction exercises. Cut out any foods that can cause bloating and make sure you drink plenty of water.

Just because there is no IBS cure it doesn't mean that you have to let it ruin your life. Get a natural colon cleanser and use it regularly. Learn what your triggers are and try your best to avoid them. You can live a normal life with IBS.

# CHAPTER 8- CAN IBS BE MISDIAGNOSED?

Irritable bowel syndrome is the most commonly diagnosed disorder by gastroenterologist. Although not everyone is diagnosed by gastroenterologists, many are diagnosed by regular physicians. There can be an error on their part when it comes to diagnosing irritable bowel syndrome. The tricky thing about irritable bowel syndrome is that there are no physical signs. When a physician or gastroenterologist comes to diagnosing possible IBS there are many things that come in to play:

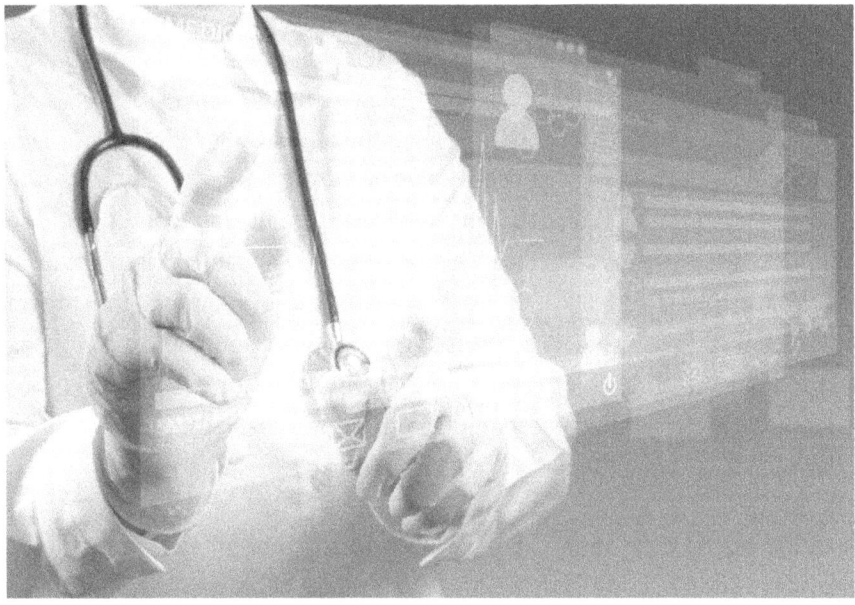

- Blood tests
- Stool sample
- Sigmoidoscopy
- Colonoscopy

## Symptoms

Without proper steps to diagnosis you can easily be diagnosed wrongly. Since there are no physical signs of IBS these above tests can rule out possible disorders with similar symptoms. Other disorders with similar symptoms are:

- Crohn's disease
- Ulcerative colitis
- Cancer (usually age 40+)
- Collagenous colitis
- Lymphocytic colitis

Plus others related to abdominal pain or bowel habit changes

If you are diagnosed with irritable bowel syndrome and actually have one of these disorders or disease you could be prolonging your pain. The common theme of these disorders is abdominal pain. Irritable bowel syndrome though doesn't have all the same treatments as the others because it is so unique. When wrongly diagnosed you could be missing out on actual sure thing cures that have been introduced to other disorders. Many of these other disorders have prescriptions that have proven to heal while IBS has a low success rate.

Irritable bowel syndrome can actually lead to some of the above listed disorders so it is important to find out exactly what you suffer from in order to set up a recovery program which will lower your chance of developing further issues.

Curing any disease is the #1 goal of anyone who suffers from one. For patients who suffer from any of the above disease, not only irritable bowel syndrome, the fastest way to end digestive pain forever is a source that presents extremely valuable information about healing and curing whatever symptoms you experience. Do not let your suffering continue, find out exactly what disorder you suffer from and treat is accordingly. If there is any sign of doubt in you irritable bowel syndrome diagnosis it can't hurt to get yourself tested again.

# ABOUT THE AUTHOR

David P Fry has been struggling with IBS for years and it was a lot of research and working along with doctors that made him find out that if the diet was adjusted that he would fare much better in the long run. As David is fully aware of the ups and downs that come with irritable bowel syndrome, he has made it his duty to speak to groups of persons that have IBS and to share his story with them.

From the information that he has garnered from his talks he managed to put a book together that would help others to learn what they really want to know about IBS.

www.ingramcontent.com/pod-product-compliance
Lightning Source LLC
Chambersburg PA
CBHW060442290526
45793CB00002B/538